BREASTFEEDING YOUR BABY: THE RIGHT CHOICE

IT JUST MAKES SENSE

GRETCHEN SLINKER JONES

BREASTFEEDING YOUR BABY:
THE RIGHT CHOICE

IT JUST MAKES SENSE

ISBN-13: 978-1456473099
ISBN-10: 1456473093
Breastfeeding Your Baby: The Right Choice
© Gretchen Slinker Jones 2010

Cover photo "Ry"©TSaltzman2008

NESTLING

For Shane & Tyler

An impatient soul
in close, dark nest suspended
twice approached me.
Communicating silently
he reached out
through the timeless void.

The essence of him
touched my heart
and loosed a quiet yearning
as the cadence
of his heartbeat spoke
in muted, magic tones.

Fraught with pain,
both his and mine,
his coming
has awakened in me
something unimagined
even in my wildest dreams.

His journey at an end,
a heretofore unknown
perception of mortality he brings;
this warm and wondrous
life creation
here embodied – infant son.

Nestling©1989 Gretchen Slinker Jones

Introduction

This updated volume has been created to replace the original, *Breastfeeding: A Mother's Guide.*

If you are seriously reading this book and did not just pick it up from somebody's coffee table, you probably recently found out you are pregnant and are researching a variety of baby- and pregnancy-related subjects.

If this is your first pregnancy, your life has changed in a way that is both terrifying and exciting. Bringing a child into the world is a big responsibility with big rewards, as well as big challenges.

As the birth of your baby approaches, your life turns into a constant stream of decisions and choices, from "necessity" choices such as picking out your crib, car seat, changing table, swing, mobiles and toys to major decisions such as whether you should use Lamaze instead of delivery drugs or breast milk instead of formula.

Let me state up front that I never intentionally set out to write a book on breastfeeding. This book is one of those things that "just happens" to people who write. The thoughts start flowing and the next thing you know, there it is — a book on whatever subject!

The basic concepts included in this text were originally self-published in 1984 and revised in 1989 after my second son was a toddler, then subsequently published under the title *Breastfeeding: A Mother's Guide* in 2009. It became obvious this year that an additional update and overhaul was genuinely justified.

Centuries ago, breastfeeding babies was not a choice, it was how babies were fed. In the late 1800s, an option to not breastfeed children was developed, commercially produced and marketed. Was this a good thing or a bad thing, overall? I am not qualified to speculate. Undoubtedly, the development of infant formula saved the lives of many infants worldwide. Whether this "miracle development" created more problems than it solved will be debated for decades.

With an increased awareness of the potential hazards of today's packaging (plastic and other types) and preservatives, not to mention possible contaminants (either intentional or unintentional) from factory production processes, more and more women are choosing to "go natural" and give their babies the best "formula" ever created — breast milk.

Please note that I am not a medical practitioner in any sense of the term and you should not interpret anything I write as "medical advice." Your doctor or midwife should be your primary source of information on all subjects having to do with your pregnancy and your baby.

What you will find in this book is a mother's insight on what worked for her.

What you will not find in this book is endless, perhaps questionable, studies and statistics to further confuse you.

This book is intended to supplement other information you will be reading during this time and offer you the one "strategy" that made a huge difference in my successful breastfeeding experience [Chapter 8].

Because I honestly believe it could make the difference between success and failure for some of those who read it and take it to heart, I am convinced it is important to share my experience with others.

Breastfeeding is important enough to our children to justify my time and effort in getting this book back into circulation to be shared.

Whether or not you breastfeed your

babies is a decision that can and should be made together by both the soon-to-be mother and the soon-to-be father, with the advice of their doctor and/or other medical practitioner. However, the physiological commitment is ultimately made by the mother-to-be and the factors of her overall health and lifestyle should be the deciding factors in all cases.

Gretchen Slinker Jones

TABLE OF CONTENTS

Breastfeeding Your Baby: The Right Choice

THE RIGHT CHOICE, THE ONLY CHOICE

Breastfeeding Your Baby: The Right Choice

1

Let's not waste any time getting to the topic at hand. That is, after all, what we are all "here" for. In my humble opinion, breastfeeding is the only choice for any mother capable of undertaking it. You cannot get any more direct than that!

Obviously, I have my reasons for being so adamant about this topic, and I will explain all of them in varying amounts of detail to you in the pages that follow. You probably agree with the general concept of breastfeeding your baby — or are at least very seriously thinking about it — or you would not have purchased this book.

Do not misunderstand, I do realize that not every woman, even in our modern world, can successfully breastfeed a baby — for a variety of reasons — including: (1) Mom is working part-time or full-time (whether by choice or by necessity) and has been unsuccessful using a breast pump for adequate quantities of milk, or (2) A medical practitioner has confirmed genuine medical reasons of one sort or another why breastfeeding is not going to be a possibility for Mom and baby at this time.

But I also believe, both from researching the subject and from the experiences of people I know personally, that many women are inaccurately told they "can't" breastfeed when they actually CAN — and that, in my opinion, is a real shame.

In fact, it would not surprise me if the majority of the women who have been influenced to believe they could not or should not breastfeed, regardless of the motives behind the influence, actually could have done so — or could have continued longer, if they for whatever reason "had to quit" earlier than they had initially planned or hoped for.

As I have listened to stories of failed attempts at breastfeeding told by women of all ages and backgrounds over the last 25+ years, I have come to a pretty clear understanding of the issues that commonly influence success or failure. Many of them are lifestyle choices. Some of them are genuine physiological difficulties. More than a few are situations where I believe success could have been ultimately achieved with adequate information and an extra measure of persistence.

Some women who could more than likely breastfeed successfully are foiled by simple circumstances that can be easily changed in many cases. Too many women either give up too quickly or start into the venture with the attitude that the attempt will fail — and, no surprise, it does fail.

As I prepared to give birth the first time, at the more-than-mature age of 28, I read everything I could get my hands on about breastfeeding. There were many, many books available, even in 1983 — at the library, in bookstores, and on the bookshelves of friends and relatives (and via the Lamaze class instructor).

Although there was no doubt in my own mind that breastfeeding was the path I wanted to follow, it was my desire to tap every source of information I could so that I would have the best possible chance to succeed. More than just a few women in my circle of friends and relatives had NOT had success nursing some or all of their children and were happy to share their stories of failure; but I did not, at any point, consider feeding infant formula to either of my sons.

It may not be possible, but please try to avoid spending a lot of time around people who speak negatively about breastfeeding, either regarding their own experiences or relating stories of someone else's experiences. Too much "exposure" to negativity can eventually erode your confidence.

There are so many books and sources of information on breastfeeding available now (including literally tens of thousands of sources online) that a person could not begin to read all of them. You will have to pick and choose, not only what you read, but what you believe.

You may have already read half a dozen books on pregnancy and breastfeeding, which is perfectly acceptable. Filter the information through what you already know and understand, and you will be able to come up with a knowledge base that should carry you through to success.

What follows in the rest of this book is a summary of the primary reasons I felt so strongly about my own personal choice and continue to advocate breastfeeding as the logical, responsible choice for moms everywhere. I could go on and on expressing my views about this subject, but I will keep it to a few main points that I believe are critical to making an informed choice and to success, which is the ultimate goal for all of us.

For the benefit of the "average reader" who has probably already spent more than a little time "studying" the information available on this subject, I have tried to be "conversational" rather than "clinical" in my approach to writing; and my sincere hope is that you will be able to take enough away from what you have read here to be more confident that you can succeed in breastfeeding your baby than you were when you started reading this book.

The reasons against feeding infant formula, even part time, vastly outnumber the reasons for it, in my humble opinion. Unless a mother is seriously malnourished or has verified health complications that make it unadvisable (either for her own health or the health of the baby), virtually all mothers should be able to successfully breastfeed for as long as they deem appropriate for their child.

Normal breast milk, from the delivery room forward, contains everything a human infant needs to not only survive, but thrive in the first several months of life.

And beyond the aspect of nutrition, breastfeeding is beneficial for the physical and emotional well being of both the mother and the child. Breastfeeding your child is a gift — and most important of all, it is absolutely the way God meant it to be.

YET YOU BROUGHT ME
OUT OF THE WOMB;
YOU MADE ME TRUST IN
YOU EVEN AT MY
MOTHER'S BREAST.
~ PSALM 22:9 ~

PORTABLE 24/7/365 EVERYWHERE

2

One Hundred Percent Portability

Breast milk is without a doubt THE only 100% portable food for babies. Feeding breast milk does not require you to provide a carrying case, a heat source, or a container from which to either dispense or consume it. It will not spoil (except in very rare cases), and there are no circumstances in which it will be the wrong temperature for your baby to consume night or day, winter or summer, indoors or outdoors.

When my oldest son was born, we lived in a rural area 17 miles from the nearest town (the last two miles were a dirt road) and 26 miles from the 2nd nearest town, so car trips for shopping, doctor visits (in the 2nd town), eating out, and virtually all other personal and family activities involved a minimum of half an hour of traveling time each way, depending on the season of the year and the weather. This was in Alaska, so winter driving conditions could continue up to 6½ months of the year, making a long trip to "town" even longer.

Although I suppose there may have been products available at the time to keep a bottle of formula from freezing in a car parked in front of a store for an hour at -30º or -40º, it would have been inconvenient, to say the least, to deal with bottles of infant formula away from home in winter in Alaska. I gave birth to babies in November and December, so obviously, keeping formula from freezing in an automobile would have been an unavoidable issue for me for at least the first few months of my boys' lives.

Our family's winter activities included ice fishing, riding ATVs and snowmachines, and attending frigid outdoor activities such as the Anchorage Fur Rendezvous and the starting ceremonies of the Iditarod sled dog race. I cannot imagine any circumstance in which it would have been possible to bottle feed a baby outdoors during any of those activities. Breastfeeding a baby snuggled into a front pack inside a big down coat in the most severe cold was no problem, however.

Our summer and fall lifestyles were full

Breastfeeding Your Baby: The Right Choice

of fishing, hunting, riding ATVs, and tent camping. None of those activities included refrigeration. Water had to be carried in containers. Space for "stuff" was limited in boats and backpacks and on the racks of a 4-wheeler.

Had I been formula-feeding my babies, it would have come down to a choice between participating in these activities with the rest of my family or staying at home with a baby alone (or worse, insisting that the rest of the family stay home with me since I could not go). What kind of choice is that? None at all, if you ask me!

With breastfeeding, there was no need to make such a choice. I am so very grateful for having had the option to be a full participant. Based on my family lifestyle, my enjoyment of living would have been much diminished while raising babies had I not been able to breastfeed them.

As moms, we sometimes have to make sacrifices to achieve what is best for our children, but giving up family time or enjoyable activities because formula feeding will not "fit" into the activity should not be one of those sacrifices.

You, of course, have to set your own priorities and make your own choices based on your family's lifestyle and your personal convictions. My family priorities may not be the same as yours. 24/7/365 portability was only one factor in the decision-making process for my family.

◆ ◆ ◆ ◆

Wardrobe Wants and Needs

The days of having to "bare yourself" in public to nurse your baby are, thankfully, long past. Today, the wardrobe of a nursing mother can not only be stylish and truly "trendy," but can be as extensive and impressive as you choose or can afford.

If you witness a mother being immodest in the public nursing of her baby today, it is because the opinion of anyone else on the subject does not concern her, not because she does not have an alternate choice in her means and methods.

If you have Internet access, a simple search for "nursing blouse," "nursing clothing" or "nursing dress" will provide a tremendous variety of choices for building a wardrobe or for gathering ideas to make your own similar clothing (or have them custom made for you by a seamstress).

Consignment shops and stores that sell used maternity clothing and baby supplies are easily found in most cities, if you are on a tight budget. Some churches operate used-clothing shops that give away items at no cost if your budget is "beyond tight."

In the months preceding the birth of my first son (1983), my mother, an accomplished seamstress, volunteered to design a whole wardrobe of "nursing" blouses and nightgowns for me, ranging from floor-length flannel gowns (for cold Alaska winter nights) to Western-yoked casual shirts, to frilly summer blouses. Mom had seen nursing garments somewhere and had bought a pattern. Because she had a talent and a gift for adapting and designing patterns, Mom created her own "signature" line of custom clothing, just for me. What a fabulous nursing wardrobe I had!

Some of the blouses were very casual, others were extravagantly "dressy" — some were heavy winter garments and others were light summer clothes. Part of them had Velcro™ enclosures and others had zippers. All of them served their purpose and enabled me to modestly nurse anytime and anywhere "in public" through two babies four years apart.

It is difficult to express what an incredible blessing it was to have these wardrobe options created by the hands of a loving "grandma-to-be" (she had lots of other grandchildren preceding mine).

Although I consider the "nursing blouse" to be an ingenious creation (and I do not know who originally created it), both Velcro™ fasteners and zippers had their minor "downsides." All things considered, though, both of these closure options worked quite nicely.

Velcro™ can get caught in long hair (I started braiding my hair at that time) or in a soft baby blanket. It is significantly destructive to chenille fabrics, so be careful. Velcro™ can be easier to open and close with one hand, however, depending on where you are sitting, standing or walking as you nurse. Velcro™ can be a better option for getting a quick, discrete closure in a public place.

Zippers often take two hands, and sometimes getting them zipped and unzipped is hard to accomplish while holding onto a wiggly baby. Zippers, however, for the most part, provide a more secure closure than Velcro™, which can come unfastened fairly easily in some circumstances, especially as it gets "older."

Keep in mind that you will have to closely monitor where your baby's face rests in relation to either a zipper or Velcro™. Both closure options can have a painful and undesirable effect on a baby's tender skin after just a few moments of direct contact. You will have to experiment a bit to see how to protect your baby from both types of closures as you nurse.

Several years after my mom crafted her creations on my behalf, there were many such items available "ready-made" in stores to enable nursing mothers to modestly feed their babies almost anywhere. "Necessity is the mother of invention" is definitely the rule here. As more and more women ended up outside their own home for extended periods of time (either working or undertaking recreational activities) while their babies were nursing, solutions obviously had to be found to meet this new clothing market demand.

Nursing moms today have almost

unlimited nursing-garment choices that include halters and hoodies, dresses and swimsuits, wraps and tanks. What a difference 25 years makes!

◆ ◆ ◆ ◆

A Public Display?

A couple of decades ago, I felt compelled to write a letter to the editor of our regional newspaper in answer to a published editorial piece complaining about a young woman who had been observed nursing her infant in the front pew of a church.

Although I have to agree that her choice of the front pew was probably not the best location for this activity; I personally believe I would much rather see the young woman in church with her baby listening to the sermon, if that is what she needed at the time, than to have her miss out on a blessing or inspiration because somebody — anybody — might be offended by something so natural as a mother feeding her baby.

The editorial in question indicated that the woman was not in any way immodest in her actions. The writer simply thought it to be inappropriate use of a church pew. His opinion was that she should have stayed home with her baby until the child was weaned. This was not an uncommon viewpoint at that time, and the issue still comes up occasionally today.

Many churches (and other places, including malls and office buildings) in our modern world have thoughtfully provided quiet, comfortable areas specifically designed for nursing mothers. And more and more states are actually passing legislation dealing with a mother's right to nurse her child in public without being accused of (and facing legal consequences for) "flashing" anybody or "indecent exposure." Who would have imagined that such amenities would ever be available? I would love to have been the individual who patented the "baby changing stations" that you see in public restrooms virtually everywhere you go today.

There are, without a doubt, locations and situations where nursing really should not take place. I observed a classic one not very long before this book was published. And it was not at all because the mother was being immodest in her behavior, it was because the baby did not have a ghost of a chance to concentrate on nursing in the stands at a riotously noisy college basketball game.

This young mother, who obviously did not have a clue, was doing her baby a disservice. And, sadly, the two-week old infant came away from the attempted feeding hungry and frustrated — and justifiably so.

Please keep in mind that babies can keep their attention on only one thing at a time — and especially when they are very young, they have to focus seriously on suckling and nothing else.

As an adult, I have a hard time focusing on anything in the stands at a college basketball game. The noise level, bright lights, and crowded conditions create an environment that is a recipe for failure to attempt to nurse a baby. It should be "common sense," but people do not always consider such things, especially if this is their first child.

With some babies, any distraction — even a seemingly minor one — can have an adverse effect on whether the suckling is successful and the baby receives adequate nutrition and/or is satisfied. This is one of the reasons why breastfeeding is sometimes not successful. The baby is too often not given an opportunity to fully concentrate on the task at hand.

Especially when your baby is very young, you may have to make difficult choices and curtail or eliminate some of your own activities to give your baby the best possible opportunity to receive critical nutrition. This is not an area for compromise. This is IMPORTANT!

There are, indeed, some babies who are much more tolerant, especially as they get a little older. You are the "expert" on your baby. It is up to you to critically observe how noise, light and motion affect your baby's focus on nursing and take appropriate action to make sure you do not inadvertently impede your baby's ability to take in nourishment (and your ability to successfully breastfeed for the long-term).

There may be occasions when your baby's developing body has decided it is feeding time and you are not anywhere near a quiet place. You will have to do your best in such an unforeseen circumstance. Covering your baby's head with a blanket (safely with enough air to breathe, of course) and/or covering his or her "exposed" ear with your hand can help, but is not always enough. One of your baby's ears will generally already be at least partially covered, snuggled up against your body.

Your baby's tolerance of light and noise may change from time to time, so always make sure you are aware of how your baby is reacting and take appropriate action or modify your activities for a time, if necessary.

Making a hungry baby wait for any length of time for you to get to a quiet place to nurse (or feed with a bottle, for that matter) is ill advised. An agitated or frustrated baby is less likely to be able to successfully take in adequate nutrition. It is important for you to do your best to anticipate when your baby might need feeding, and try to schedule your events and activities to accommodate your baby's needs — this is "priority one" during the time period in your life that you are breastfeeding. It is part of the "sacrifice," and it is absolutely worth it.

My first breastfeeding "adventure"

included nursing my first-born son in a Gerry™ front pack while touring Ghirardelli Square in San Francisco when he was seven weeks old. A light blanket over the baby's head and my shoulder, and "voila" — lunch is served at the "mobile street café"! On that particular trip, he also nursed in a wax museum, my brother's Volkswagen "bug," on the "Bart" train, at the zoo, and in an Oriental restaurant (Speaking from personal experience, I would advise against eating with chopsticks and a baby in your lap).

Unfortunately, there is always someone who will find fault with the idea of nursing babies "in public." Frankly, I doubt that any of the people I encountered had the slightest inkling of what was going on when I nursed my son while strolling down the sidewalks of San Francisco. I might just as easily have been covering the baby's head to keep the chill of the ocean breeze away from him. No one could tell he was "dining."

During his first ten months of life, my firstborn was modestly nursed in malls, airports, cars, restaurants, homes of friends and relatives, boats — and even on a parked snowmachine. The noise of the snowmachine engine turned out to be bothersome to my babies, so I did have to discontinue that activity while my children were small.

Both of my sons experienced trips to Disneyland in their early lives — and riding in a backpack hiking on sand dunes — and watching sled dog competitions in Alaska. No matter where or when the "hungries" occurred, the supply was always available, and always ready to serve. Who could ask for anything more?

♦ ♦ ♦ ♦

Long-Distance Travel

Because we lived 3,000 miles from most of our relatives, family visits during our "baby days" involved long airplane trips with a never-ending variety of transitions from airplane to airplane and layovers of varying lengths. Flight complications thrown in by fog, ice, and totally-unanticipated circumstances, such as an airline hostess strike, can make instantly available baby food even more valuable and appreciated!

There is no more perfect way to feed a baby on an airplane or in an airport waiting area than nursing. In addition, I had read — and my own experience confirmed it over and over again — that nursing an infant on an airplane was an excellent way to help stabilize the baby's ears when the plane was taking off and landing. I am pleased to report that I did not ever have any issues with a baby screaming because his ears were in pain, because I nursed my "babe in arms" on take off and landing on every flight — and there were many flights.

Advocates of forcing parents to buy a ticket for their under-two-years-old child's car seat for domestic flights have, to date, been unsuccessful, although the subject does still come up now and then. It is true that in an airplane crash, an infant would probably be safer strapped into a car seat; however, there really are so few crashes compared to the number of people flying and the number of trips flown, that it is probably not an issue that would save a significant number of lives. Airplane crashes, more often than not, are so severe that car seats may or may not make any difference at all in potential for survival of an "under-two."

Beyond the obvious cost of a ticket for the seat, an infant strapped into a car seat next to your airplane seat would probably be screaming the whole time the plane was taking off and landing. For safety reasons, it would be unlikely that parents (or baby) would be allowed to have a baby bottle in hand and not "stored" away during takeoff and landing. So there could be no relief for baby's ears from suckling, even a bottle, in that scenario. We will hope, for the sake of the babies, that the advocates of buckling infants into car seats on domestic airplane flights do not ever succeed in their efforts to change policies.

It is debatable whether sucking on a pacifier (if the baby will take one, mine would not) helps the ears on an airplane. It might be better than nothing, however, if that was your only choice when flying with your infant or toddler.

And to say that parents should just stay home instead of traveling on airplanes with small children is ridiculous. We are not even going to go there! Families are spread across the country — and sometimes the world — today. There is not much we can do about it, and extended airplane travel is an inevitable "fact of life" for many families.

Although older children and adults can chew gum, this is not even remotely

Breastfeeding Your Baby: The Right Choice

possible for the very young. Those who complain about crying babies on planes often lack information and compassion. Who can blame infants for loudly protesting pain they are experiencing? Babies whose ears hurt do not have any alternative to complaining. It is not as if they are purposely trying to irritate the other passengers on the airplane. Babies are not making their own ears hurt! People cannot expect them to act like they are not babies — they ARE babies! What a ridiculous notion.

The nursing baby, unless there are other issues with ears or sinuses, rarely has any difficulty with airplane take off and landing times.

I do strongly recommend that women flying alone with an "under-two" have a front carrier or sling of some sort, even for a child you would not normally carry in one, just so you can safely nap (or rest your arms) if your little one falls asleep in your lap while nursing during a long flight.

Between weather delays, equipment malfunctions, and stewardess strikes, there were several occasions when I was stuck in an airport with a baby for many, many hours longer than originally planned. Having the ability to nurse anytime, anywhere was a genuine lifesaver for both me and the baby in those unforeseen and unfortunate situations.

♦ ♦ ♦ ♦

And Then There Was Night

Finally, the ultimate "portability" aspect of nursing a baby pertains to nighttime feedings.

Today, moms may choose to have their baby right next to them in a mattress-level crib open on the "bed" side and nurse at any time during the night that the baby is hungry. Baby has his or her own "space," but there is no barrier between baby and Mom (or Dad). I would love to have had a "cool tool" like that when my boys were infants! If such a thing was available at the time, I had not been made aware of it. The first time I personally saw one was in 2001.

Breastfeeding at night, to me, meant not getting out of a warm bed to be blinded by lights or thump and bump your way down the hall in the near-dark to the kitchen to prepare formula. The only exception to this was in times of major milk-production spurts when I needed to use a warm washcloth to get the milk flowing well, and I DID have to get out of the bed to get the warm washcloth when my husband was out of town working and was not available to do it for me.

No heating up bottles, no parents trying to get back to much-needed sleep, no hungry baby frustrated with waiting for the bottle to get "made" and then having trouble nursing because his whole digestive system was understandably upset by what I refer to as the "waaaa-waiting syndrome."

Does this sound like a sweet deal to you? I certainly found it to be so sweet I would not have given it up for anything or anyone.

My personal experience was that once the baby was finished nursing, both my baby and I went right back to sleep until the next feeding (with both of my boys). I know that there are many who argue you should not sleep with your baby in your bed; but in more than four years of feedings, I never had any difficulty or experienced anything I ever perceived to be a dangerous situation. Frequently the baby never made it back into the bedside cradle — both he and I often fell asleep during the nursing process.

There are wonderful options today for your baby to be almost in the bed with you, but still safely separate. You and your husband, along with your doctor or midwife, can discuss this safety issue and come up with a solution that fits your family's needs and wants.

Search online for "bedside sleeper" or "bedside crib" and you will come up with most, if not all, of the choices available. Make sure you purchase a product made by a reputable company. Check for recalls. And if you decide to purchase a used item, get the model number and check out the consumer safety status before buying.

Take note that I am not advocating for parents to sleep with a baby in their bed — there are MANY who caution against it, for obvious reasons. This is a personal choice that each family has to make after gathering enough information to make a decision that works for them and their household.

◆ ◆ ◆ ◆

Summing It Up

Breast milk is available 24/7/365; and

no matter where you are, you should be able to find an appropriate place to stop what you are doing and feed your baby.

"Mommy milk" is always the right temperature, and it does not have any additives or preservatives unless your diet is so riddled with them that they work their way into your milk. Most nursing moms are very conscious of what they eat and drink, so excessive amounts of additives and preservatives are not generally a problem.

Whether you are in the comfort of your own home — or at Disneyland or Atlantic City, in a boat on the river or on a tram at the ski resort, at the park or the pool, you are always ready to nourish your child at a moment's notice. Who would not find that desirable?

ENVIRONMENTALLY FRIENDLY "PACKAGING"

Breastfeeding Your Baby: The Right Choice

3

Plastics and Non-Renewable Resources

No one can convincingly argue against the fact that the packaging breast milk comes in (in virtually all cases) is non-toxic, natural, "organic," and environmentally friendly. No waste, no use of non-renewable resources, no toxic inks, no plastic "blister packs." The evidence is simply indisputable.

We all know that it takes both "fuel" and "materials" — many of them non-renewable resources — to get infant formula manufactured, into the package and delivered to the store shelf. Between coated metal or cardboard cans and plastic containers, there is a tremendous amount of "manufacturing" involved in production of infant formula, plus transportation of goods both before and after the packaging.

Baby bottles are almost all plastic these days — and although there are new developments being made with alternate substances, the majority of plastics are still produced from petroleum. The majority of plastics are also produced in foreign countries, with varying amounts of safety regulation, and transported to the United States for purchase and use by people who may not even be aware of the source of the product, or the safety or quality of the manufacturing process.

Our country's addiction to plastics is one of the primary reasons we are so dependent on "foreign oil." It makes sense that nursing your baby will contribute, in at least a small way, to reducing our dependence on production of more plastics and packaging materials from petroleum.

Even glass bottles use resources — including hot water (most commonly heated by electricity or natural gas) and soap (perhaps not environmentally safe) to sanitize them — and create waste that has to be disposed of, as well as detergents and cleaning solutions that go down your drains and out into a waste treatment plant or septic system. Even the act of boiling water on the stove (or using the sterilization setting on your dishwasher) consumes energy resources, when you get right down to it.

"Blister packs" developed for convenient display on store shelves, plus racks for nipples, pacifiers, teething rings and other potentially-harmful baby "accessories" use huge amounts of plastics, inks, and cardboard when you lump them all together, as well. Wow! What a waste!

If you spend five minutes looking around the baby section in any store, you can clearly see both the environmental and the financial bottom-line "cost" of plastic and cardboard packaging and the plastic or synthetic products inside the packaging.

If this element of the discussion is not important to you, you can skip on to the next chapter of the book. We do not all think alike — and we shouldn't. That is one of the beauties of a free society!

Although some nursing moms will use bottles part of the time, there are many nursing mothers who never even purchase a single baby bottle.

◆ ◆ ◆ ◆

Environmental Waste

The amount of environmental waste

created by the production, packaging, and distribution of infant formula, baby bottles, and artificial nipples is absolutely staggering.

Admittedly, production, packaging and disposal of "nursing bras" and disposable nursing pads does use some resources and create some waste. You will obviously have to weigh the pros and cons of the environmental impact of these items and make your decisions on purchasing them based on the facts and your own personal situation and circumstances.

Recycling of glass and plastic sometimes consumes more non-renewable resources than it saves by the time waste is transported by truck or rail (consuming large quantities of fossil fuels) to a recycling facility, after which the recycling machinery is operated to complete the process and the end products are trucked (or transported by train or plane) to wherever the recycled products are "reused."

Fortunately, newer and better waste management techniques are coming into play and will continue to do so in the foreseeable future. But waste disposal is still a critical issue that we must consider.

Don't get me started about the waste created by manufacture and use of disposable diapers! The data on that issue is mind boggling. I do not see how we can continue to use disposable diapers at the rate we are currently using them and survive the mountains of waste that are being created day in and day out, year after year, both in America and around the world!

I will talk more about disposable diapers versus cloth later on.

Breastfeeding Your Baby: The Right Choice

A
REASONABLY-PRICED
"PRODUCT"

Breastfeeding Your Baby: The Right Choice

4

The Financial Side of "Mommy Milk" vs. Infant Formula

Maybe you have more money than we did, but I cannot imagine being a new parent and spending all of the money required to feed a child from newborn infant through 100% solid food in this day and age with products not from "Mom."

Even if you are able to purchase infant formula "on sale," with coupon discounts, or at discount or warehouse food outlets, buying formula is still a tremendous expense — and sometimes can even be a serious financial burden — on an already stretched-tight family budget following the long list of expenses involved with the delivery of babies (even if everything goes perfectly) and the purchase of all of the furniture, clothing and additional supplies required — or desired — to bring a new baby home.

Unanticipated complications to a pregnancy or delivery can change the financial balance from "ok" to "oh no!" in a matter of moments, hours or days. Such circumstances can be the deciding factor for some families in whether or not to breastfeed their baby, although I believe finances should never be the only reason to make the decision to breastfeed.

With the exception of nursing bras and nursing pads, there should be virtually no "have to" cost involved with breastfeeding your baby. You should be consuming nutritious food to rebuild your post-partum body, regardless of whether or not you are nursing your baby, so quality food cannot realistically count as an "expense" related to breastfeeding.

Check around for affordable sources for nursing bras. You may be able to use them through nursing of multiple children, so it will not necessarily be an expense associated with every pregnancy and birth. If you have a consignment shop or used clothing store you trust, you can probably buy nursing bras with a relatively small "investment." Some women, under-standably, prefer not to purchase and wear undergarments that have been worn by someone else, even for a short time.

There are several available choices for "non-disposable" nursing pads. And how extensively you use them (either disposable or not) will be determined somewhat by how much you are away from home or entertaining guests during the times when your milk production is in "overflow" stage.

If you decide to take advantage of nursing garments, there will obviously be a cost for the purchase of those items (unless you have a mother like mine who just makes them and gives them to you). There are second-hand stores in every city that specialize in gently-used pre- and post-pregnancy clothing items and baby items, so you may not have to buy new unless you particularly want to. It is highly likely that these items will last you through more than one child, however, minimizing the cost.

◆ ◆ ◆ ◆

The Transition to "Real Food"

Once your baby is able to begin consuming soft "real" foods, you can also save money by making your own "baby food." I personally did not feed my boys anything — even baby crackers or jarred cereal — until after they were three or four months old and very little in the way of "food" until they were 12 months of age. (This was with the wholehearted support of my pediatrician.)

Regular checkups, along with your own observations, will determine whether your baby is receiving adequate nutrition from breast milk alone. And remember, that any "food" you give your baby will eventually reduce your milk supply. As you work into soft foods, this will naturally occur as part of the eventual weaning process.

With the help of your doctor or midwife and other available resources, your family will have to make a choice on when to begin feeding foods other than breast milk. There are many sources of information available, so take advantage of them.

I would guess these days that most people already own some sort of food processor, unless they do not have electricity (we still have folks in our rural area that do NOT have electricity in their homes in 2010). For "unplugged" folks, there are a number of choices of hand grinders available.

In 1983, when I gave birth to son #1, we did not own a food processor; so after researching what was available and what would do the job for us, we bought a Cuisinart™ "pro" model. We still use it in 2010, at the time of the 2nd revision to this book, though not for babies as my "baby" is over 23 at the time of this writing. The old Cuisinart™ is still useful for producing "baby food" when our grandkids are visiting, however. There are many new choices for processing home-made "baby food," including mini-choppers that make one serving at a time for ultimate freshness.

It is common "wisdom" that you should introduce just one food item at a time to your baby. I followed this advice faithfully, and neither of my boys has ever had any kind of food allergy, all the way from birth to adulthood. Take your time. There is no reason to hurry in getting new foods introduced to a baby.

When making your own "baby food," avoid highly seasoned foods and refined sugars, if possible. Natural is best. If you can afford them, I would shop for organic fruits, vegetables, and meats as a precaution against toxins and/or steroids.

Potentially harmful food sources are much more prevalent today than they were when I had babies!

There is really no need to add seasonings at all when preparing baby foods. If your little one will eat completely unseasoned food and enjoy it, let him develop a taste for FOOD, not seasonings. Carrots are naturally sweet, and so are sweet potatoes and yams. Fruit by itself is very tasty. As with food for adults, think in terms of: the more brightly colored the food, the more nutritious it usually is.

Just think how much more money you will have available to spend on other things — whether they be "necessities" or "frills" — if you are producing your own baby foods from items you already have in your house, some of which you are cooking for your own meals. It just makes sense!

You could probably take a vacation on the money saved by not buying infant formula and baby food for a year. Who could argue that is not a "bargain" worth making a small sacrifice to get?

WHOLESOME
VS.
POTENTIALLY TOXIC

Breastfeeding Your Baby: The Right Choice

5

What's In YOUR Bottle?

As more and more information is available on just what goes into products that come from factories — whether in or out of the United States — it appears abundantly clear to me that breast milk is truly the only "natural" solution to feeding your child, especially in the critical early infant stage.

Credible news reports have brought to light serious issues with some of the properties of plastic bottles, including some baby bottles (reportedly perhaps as many as 95% of them), and "sippy cups," as well as some artificial nipples and pacifiers.

BPA (Bisphenol A) has been reported by numerous sources and agencies as being potentially dangerous to humans (both adults and children), and this toxin can be found in other baby-related items such as teething rings and toys that a baby will frequently put in his or her mouth. A web search will provide you with a number of sources of information on the topic of BPA in the plastics and resins we use today.

Until more studies are done, it is prudent to consider NOT using these products in your baby's most important growth and development stages (if ever). There is some research-based speculation that even conditions such as autism and Asperger's could be caused by BPA or other toxins in the wide variety of plastics our babies come in daily contact with from birth to age three and beyond.

There are manufacturing codes on the bottom of every bottle. Do some research to see which ones have been identified as being unsafe — and consider not using any plastic bottles at all.

Keep in mind that if you pump or express milk to be stored for your baby to consume when you are away from home or working, it should, perhaps, not be stored or served in plastic bottles. Glass bottles are still available, and they are a better choice for both storage and feeding of breast milk, if necessary. Buy them from a quality company you trust.

There is no doubt in my mind that to err on the side of safety is the appropriate course of action when it comes to plastics and toxins and your baby's life and health.

◆ ◆ ◆ ◆

Artificial/Synthetic vs. God-Designed

Artificial nipples are made from an ever-increasing variety of materials, including latex, rubber, and silicone. It has been widely speculated that artificial nipples likely contribute to development of allergies in some babies. Consider how many people today are allergic to latex. It is definitely something to think about.

By the time parents or doctors figure out a baby is allergic to certain materials, allergies can sometimes already be developed and the consequences may initiate a lifelong health battle for the individual with the allergies.

◆ ◆ ◆ ◆

Toxic Absorption

Because under the tongue is one of the places humans rapidly absorb virtually anything almost directly into the bloodstream (which is why homeopathy remedies are dispensed and dissolved under the tongue), there is considerable reason to question the safety of having a plastic nipple, pacifier or teething ring in your baby's mouth for any length of time — if ever. Is it alarmist to consider such ideas? I do not believe it is. This is our babies we are talking about!

I have observed babies (and toddlers) who have a "binkie" or "plug" in their mouth almost 24/7. It does not take much effort to calculate how many hours a two year old has had that pacifier in his or her mouth if it has been used "most" of the time since infancy.

Babies are virtually guaranteed to absorb into their bloodstreams anything that is available to be released from the objects you (or they) place in their mouths. Is it really worth taking a chance? Where do we draw the line on potential for harm?

Along this same line of thought, you should also do some research and be careful about what ends up on your skin in the way of lotions, soaps or crèmes in your breast and nipple areas. Many of these items also contain chemicals that have been identified as potentially dangerous to humans. What does not seem to harm your skin may turn out to be harmful to your baby's more sensitive system.

It is a "no-brainer" that virtually all pharmaceuticals, over-the-counter medications, and other potentially toxic substances that end up in or on your body have the potential to end up in the breast milk your baby is consuming. These can include hair dye, lipstick, nail polish, lotions, crèmes, makeup, soap, and even your laundry soap and fabric softener.

Make sure that clothes and bedding washed and dried with your laundry detergent and/or fabric softener are not creating an allergic reaction when your baby's skin touches clothing or bedding (either yours or theirs). This is something a lot of people do not take into consideration (and it is not always related to breastfeeding), but it is a valid concern.

Breastfeeding Your Baby: The Right Choice

NATURALLY NUTRITIOUS

Breastfeeding Your Baby: The Right Choice

6

Your "Diet," Your Baby's Diet

Human breast milk was designed by the Creator for human babies — whereas cow milk was designed for cow babies and goat milk was designed for goat babies. I never gave birth to any calves or kid goats, and I am sure you will not do so, either. It stands to reason that human babies should be fed human milk, and nothing but human milk, whenever it is humanly possible.

Through the early life of an infant/toddler, human breast milk automatically adjusts to the nutritional needs of the child. It contains antibodies that help an immature immune system cope with the hazardous new environment it will encounter for months and years to come.

There has reportedly been an increase in the number of women breastfeeding their babies since at least 2000. Even the World Health Organization recommends that for optimum nutrition, babies worldwide should receive mother's milk through at least the age of six months.

Store-bought infant formula contains a variety of substances, depending on the manufacturer. Most products contain milk whey and other substances to provide the "protein component," some form of vegetable oil to provide the "fat component" (yes, babies need fat in their milk), and synthetic and/or natural vitamin-mineral supplements. It is possible that there are partially-hydrogenated oils (what at our house we refer to as "white death") in some formulas. Potential risk to health and development over time? Maybe. Worth investigating? Obviously.

Unless your diet (and by "diet" I mean your overall nutritional intake, not a weight-reduction diet) is seriously deficient in some way, human breast milk is perfectly nutritious. I challenge you to find anyone who can truthfully argue with this concept. There are rare exceptions, of course.

Your overall nutrition program for the period of time during which you are nursing your child will be similar to nutrition during pregnancy. It is important that you eat a balanced diet and factor in extra calories for the baby. But do not get carried away — nursing a baby is not a license to eat anything and everything you want just because you are "feeding two."

It is critical that you consume foods from all of the recommended groups, and lots of fresh fruits and vegetables, if available and affordable. I realize there are geographic locations where fresh fruits and vegetables may be available, but may not be particularly affordable, the year around. If fresh fruits and vegetables are not available (or affordable), try to select canned products that are packed with natural juices and limited added sugar and/or salt, whenever possible.

You may have found that you were sensitive to certain foods during your pregnancy, and your baby may be sensitive to these same foods (or others) through your milk. Be aware of how your baby is reacting to your milk and look for clues about what you have consumed (in either food or drink) that may have contributed to an upset stomach or change in overall health in your baby. This is very important.

You should expect to carry a few extra

pounds during the time period when you are nursing your child. There is time enough to get back your "girlish figure" later on, and there is no reason you cannot maintain a moderate fitness routine once you are fully recovered from delivery. Face facts, your body is never going to be exactly the same again, anyway.

The health of your baby is vastly more important than you being "skinny." And most nursing mothers have pre-included this "temporary sacrifice" in their overall commitment to provide their child with a natural, healthy start in life.

Repeat after me: "It's only temporary ... it's only temporary ... it's only temporary!"

♦ ♦ ♦ ♦

Soy = "Solution" or "Problem"?

I understand (but have difficulty comprehending) that, for whatever reason, some babies cannot tolerate "real" milk in any form, including from Mom, although it escapes me why that should biologically occur in God's creation.

Soy-based infant formula has its pros and cons, like any other product. The primary 21st-century concerns with soy infant formulas recently reported have to do with how the developing baby's hormones are affected (which is why pre-menopausal, peri-menopausal, and post-menopausal women commonly use soy products for estrogen control), so I am not convinced soy products are genuinely good over the long term for human babies.

Please take the time to do some research on your own, talk to your medical practitioner, and carefully consider the pros and cons before you supplement your breast milk with infant formula that contains soy products (or soy milk).

In the interest of controlling how much soy estrogen ends up in your breast milk, if you eat soy products or drink soy milk during pregnancy and nursing, bear in mind that it has the potential to have an effect on both you and your child. This is a matter that should be discussed at length with your doctor or midwife.

◆ ◆ ◆ ◆

And What About That Water Issue?

My in-laws thought I was certifiably nuts when I declined to give my baby boys water in bottles when we visited them in

California. However, I had discussed this issue in detail with my doctor; and he had advised me that breast milk has all the "water" in it that a healthy baby needs — even in summer and even in California, except in rare circumstances.

My doctor's only caution on this issue was that we should consistently monitor the baby's stools and skin flexibility to make sure there was no hint of dehydration.

In all of our visits to southern California with nursing babies, declining to provide water from a bottle never created any adverse health issues for our babies. My in-laws were eventually convinced (by the evidence in front of them) that it was alright to not provide water in bottles. Neither of my boys drank any water until they were drinking from a sippy cup.

Each family should discuss the subject of water with their doctor, nutritionist or midwife. Not everyone shares this "no-water" philosophy, and it may not be the right choice for every situation and every family. It may not be the appropriate choice for you and your baby.

◆ ◆ ◆ ◆

To Supplement or Not to Supplement

Most physicians recommend that a pre-natal supplement be continued through the period of time that a mother is nursing.

Because the first year is so critical to healthy child development, I agree that a vitamin-mineral supplement designed for nursing mothers is advisable to achieve maximum nutritional value of the mother's milk and to protect the long-term health of the mother, as well.

I certainly would not discourage a mom who eats the ideal nutritious "diet" from abstaining from taking a supplement, though, as long as the doctor has been consulted, the baby is growing steadily and both Mom and baby continue to be healthy.

Supplements are "unnatural" in their own way, and I have always advocated getting your nutrition from "real food" when possible.

When in doubt, ask your doctor.

Breastfeeding Your Baby: The Right Choice

"ON DEMAND" NURSING STARTING AT BIRTH

7

On Demand or On Schedule?

There are always arguments for and against it, but there is absolutely no doubt in my mind that nursing on demand — that is, every time the baby indicates he or she is hungry — is the only way to go, both from the perspective of your milk production and for your baby's steady growth.

And, unless there is some compelling reason against it, this practice should begin in the birthing room and should continue throughout the nursing period. Unless your post-delivery health prevents it, you should nurse your newborn on the delivery table and on demand thereafter. If your hospital has a policy against that, I would personally recommend that you consider choosing another hospital.

The colostrum, sometimes referred to as "liquid gold," in your breasts at the time of delivery is the precursor to milk and was created by God for your baby to consume until your milk "comes in." Your body system begins developing colostrum somewhere around the fifth month of your pregnancy. It is there for a reason. Use it!

In the absence of some sort of unheard of continuous "super-supply" of milk, breastfed babies cannot be successfully nursed on a "schedule." Babies go through growth spurts unpredictably and frequently; and as a result, your milk supply will naturally go through critical "supply and demand" catch-up periods.

As far as I have been able to determine, there are no exceptions to this concept. Throughout the entire time period in which you breastfeed your child, you will experience times when your milk supply is struggling to keep up with your baby's needs. This is natural and normal.

If you nurse your baby every three or four hours on a schedule, rather than when his or her ever-changing little body is ready for "intake," the highly-sophisticated milk production plant in your body will be tricked into thinking that you do not need lots of milk and will automatically reduce production. This is a fine-tuned system, not an accidental development.

A baby must be nursed when he or she is hungry — PERIOD!

♦ ♦ ♦ ♦

"Growing Pains"

It is critical that you start, early in your pregnancy, gently conditioning your nipples for the "abuse" they will undergo. You cannot breastfeed a baby if your nipples are too sore to touch. For most women, just rolling the nipple between your fingers and very gently pulling on it (make sure you wash your hands first) will successfully condition your nipples, <u>if you start well ahead of the birth of your child</u>. This should be a gradual and always gentle process. Please do not be aggressive in trying to pre-condition your nipples because you think you started too late. Keep this conditioning process reasonable and consistent.

There are products available that will help relieve sore nipples, but there is no adequate substitute for having them conditioned and ready ahead of time.

There were times, especially with my second son, that my milk production could barely keep up with his growth spurts.

During some of these periods, most of which only lasted a few days, it seemed like he had just finished nursing and he would be hungry again — and I would be nursing again, and again. There were days (and nights) when I literally spent the majority of my time nursing him. This can be "a royal pain" for several reasons, including sore nipples. But you must stick with it! Remember, it's only temporary ... You must choose to nurse whenever the baby is hungry — even if it has only been 20 minutes since he nursed — and allow your body to catch up production to sustain your baby through a growth (and consumption) spurt. Your nipples will survive!

◆ ◆ ◆ ◆

Keeping Up With Production vs. Demand

Because your milk supply will only increase production when it gets a signal that it needs to increase production, you must keep nursing through these growth spurts so your body recognizes the need to produce more milk and subsequently steps up production as fast as it can.

The human milk production "facility" is a

wonderfully- and intricately-designed system, and we too often throw a kink into the works by failing to recognize that it can only work properly when we let it function as it was designed to. Throw human "wisdom" into the mix and we have a tendency to get things all messed up.

Failing to recognize and accommodate the "supply and demand" nature of breast milk production is a common reason why women "can't" successfully breastfeed their baby. It is the primary reason why some women fail in their breastfeeding endeavor.

It is really very simple — you take more milk out, you produce more milk. You take less milk out, you produce less milk. This is one area where a lot of women get into problems, because they do not take seriously (or fully understand) the need to keep taking more and more milk out so more and more can be produced.

If you skip feedings while you are away from your baby, even if you express or pump milk out, you are likely to experience reduced production. This is partly true because even when you believe you have expressed or pumped all milk out, you often do not, in fact, get it all. Limiting your time away from your baby, especially during growth spurts, will help you succeed for your baby's health.

Nursing a baby during growth spurts can be especially difficult if you have other children who need your attention. It is a major time commitment; and it cannot succeed if you cannot fully follow through with the commitment. It truly is worth it in the end, though.

Especially with my second son when I had some "experience under my belt," there were times, when I sensed that my baby was entering a growth spurt and my production was playing "catch-up," that I actually expressed any excess milk I could produce down the sink drain after my baby had finished nursing so that my "production plant" would be convinced it needed to continue stepping up production. If I had been keeping bottled milk for a babysitter, I could have expressed that excess milk into bottles, rather than "wasting it" in the sink.

It worked every time. My body did not fail to keep up with my baby's increased demand. I was much more aware of this with my second son, though, so I did not struggle as much keeping up with milk production during those growth spurts the second time around.

For whatever reason, I did not have much success pumping milk to be used by a babysitter in my absence, so I (by my own choice) did not spend much time away from my baby either time I was nursing. I was not especially interested in spending time away from my babies and was not very committed to pumping milk, so those were probably both contributing factors.

What a blessing to have healthy children as a result of my small sacrifice, though. There truly is no substitute.

◆ ◆ ◆ ◆

No "Bad Habits" to Break – Sweeeeet!

In the long run, expressing milk for a babysitter really did not matter in my case because neither of my boys would take a bottle, with or without breast milk in it, and with or without a Nuk™ "natural" nipple on it.

Neither of the boys ever used a pacifier, either. "Mom" was the pacifier — and it always did the trick. What a blessing to not have to break a child from either the bottle or the pacifier!

There are those who would say that popping a child on the breast every time he or she is fussy, for whatever reason, would be spoiling the child. I personally never found this to be true, and I never saw any detrimental effects as a result of the practice in my own life and with my own children. There is much to be said for the comfort of the mother's breast, even if the child is not really "nursing."

Neither of my boys was overweight or otherwise unhealthy. Neither developed any allergies. Neither developed any serious behavioral issues. The ability to shop, or rest, or have a quiet conversation without dealing with a fussy infant/toddler was incentive enough for me to use the "comfort of the mother's breast" every time I deemed it to be a useful "tool."

◆ ◆ ◆ ◆

One or Two?

Even if you think your baby has been satisfied with one breast, unless he or she totally refuses the second one, you should feed with both breasts every time. This will help keep you from being overfull (and maybe <u>painfully</u> overfull) on one side, as well as help to keep production up as the baby grows and demands more milk. A super-tight, overfull condition logically would cause production to be cut down because the body will eventually respond to the "overfull" status, especially if it is repeated often.

It has been long recommended that you rotate which breast you feed first. I stayed true to that, and it worked out very nicely for me. There may be occasions when you are tired and genuinely do not remember which breast you used first for the prior feeding. Do not "worry" about it. Just pick one and start over again. It is not likely to adversely affect either you or your child for that to happen from time to time.

There will be occasions when, for whatever reason, you are "on the fly" and you simply do not have time to nurse both breasts. You will have to use your best judgment at times like that. Just do not forget that the less you take out, the less you produce. There is no way around it. If you fail to take it all out, there will be consequences in production, sooner or later.

THE MUCH-ANTICIPATED "SECRET STRATEGY"

Breastfeeding Your Baby: The Right Choice

8

Sharing the "Secret"

In all of the reading I did on breastfeeding babies during both of my pregnancies, I never came upon the "secret" that ultimately helped me the most in successfully breastfeeding my sons. It had to have been a gift from God — there is really no other explanation for it.

This "gift" is the primary reason I decided to write this book. Nothing else I learned or tried made as much of a difference as this one small thing did in my overall breastfeeding experience with both of my sons.

One of the most frequent problems moms encounter is getting the milk to let down so the baby can consume it. You can have all the milk in the world; but if the baby cannot get it — and get all of it — it is not worth much.

Breastfeeding books contain list after list

of suggestions for how to get your milk to let down. Some of them work fairly well. Some probably do not work at all. Each mother's body is different, of course.

Especially during times when production is exceeding consumption, there can be serious issues of overfull breasts, which can compromise or inhibit the "letting down" of the milk. The solution I found is so simple!

When I was at home, or otherwise indoors where I had access to a washcloth and hot water, virtually every time I was ready to nurse my baby, I soaked a wash cloth in tap water as hot as my skin could tolerate without burning myself, twisted the bulk of the water out of it so it was not "drippy," folded it twice, and then carefully pressed it gently, but firmly, on the whole breast area of the side I was going to use first and held it there for just a few brief moments.

PLEASE NOTE — You MUST be careful not to get the cloth too hot; but it worked best for me to have it as warm as I could easily tolerate. The potential for scalding your most tender skin area will depend somewhat on the temperature of your hot tap water. DO NOT BURN YOURSELF! And be careful that the cloth does not touch your baby if you are holding him or her. What your skin will tolerate is obviously not the same as what your baby's skin will tolerate.

While you are holding the cloth against your skin, take a few deep breaths and count out at least 60 seconds. If your baby is fussing, you can softly sing out the seconds to produce a calming effect until you are ready. Try not to take any longer than necessary, so your baby does not become agitated by the wait.

Going through this process softens and relaxes the tissues and allows the milk to come down virtually effortlessly. It seems to help ALL of your milk to be available; and it also helps keep your muscles and breast tissue from being overstressed and tense. I also found that it helped the flow to not "shoot out" so fast when production was in full gear, so that it did not choke the baby.

If you get the cloth too hot initially, let it cool just enough to be comfortable. You do not want to lose too much heat or you will have to start over again, which is obviously not going to help your baby get his or her milk sooner than later. DO NOT ever heat the cloth in the microwave! Use tap water.

I do not have any "medical" evidence to back it up, but I personally believe this strategy helped keep my nipples from becoming sore, as well. The more easily your baby can get the milk, the less "wear and tear" there will be on your nipples. It just plain makes sense.

It is also conceivable that using the ultra-warm wash cloth helps keep your milk ducts clear and flowing, reducing the potential for mastitis or other infections of the "milk production system," as well.

◆ ◆ ◆ ◆

So, Is There a Downside To This?

This method does sometimes necessitate getting up from your comfortable chair or bed and warming the other breast (mostly when you are at the end of a "catch-up period") when you are ready to switch. It helps if you have someone (like your wonderful husband, perhaps, or your mom or sister) who can bring you a heated washcloth for the second breast when the time comes (or for both, so you do not have to get out of bed or your easy chair at all!).

Often, both breasts let down at the

same time, so the second one is waiting and ready when you finish feeding the first and does not need the cloth treatment. Use your judgment. You will soon come to know your own body and how it is reacting.

There may be times, though, especially when you are stretched-tight overfull, that you will still need to use the warm cloth on the second breast to ensure that your nipple does not become worn out and that all of the milk will flow out of the ducts and be available to your baby.

Please do not EVER allow your production to slow down simply because you find extra-full breasts to be painful for you. This is your baby's life and health we are talking about. The warm cloth will help you be more comfortable, help your milk be more available, and help keep your nipples from becoming sore. You can do this!

Let me be clear that it is absolutely worth the extra effort and minimal inconvenience. Using this easy and cost-free method made all the difference in the world for me (and my babies), and I have shared the concept with as many women as I could over the ensuing years in the interest of trying to make their breastfeeding experience more rewarding and successful.

I genuinely believe that if more women would try this strategy, more would experience long-term success in breastfeeding their babies. What can initially seem like a problem of supply may simply be that your milk is not getting to where your baby can get it. Frustration starts building and milk production starts plunging — and the whole experience ends up with your baby on formula. What a waste!

It might be hard to believe that such a simple solution could make that much difference. I hope that you will commit to at least trying the method (more than once) and ultimately find it to be successful. Being able to breastfeed your baby for as long as <u>you</u> choose is such a rewarding experience, for both you and your baby.

There is nothing to compare with the feeling you get when you are nursing your baby. Women who have never done it can scarcely imagine it, unfortunately. It is truly a blessing!

A QUESTION OF HOW AND WHERE

Breastfeeding Your Baby: The Right Choice

9

It's All About Comfort

One of the important factors in successfully breastfeeding your child is where you undertake this activity.

It is essential that you have a quiet, comfortable place to nurse your baby, especially during the first few days. I had a favorite recliner for both of my boys. It ended up being my younger son's favorite recliner until it finally fell apart when he was about 10 years old.

Although it might seem insignificant, it helps if you can use the same location as often as possible so the baby does not continually have "new" things to look at and be distracted by, increasing the potential for failure.

Daytime, however, will likely be different than nighttime unless your favorite recliner is in your bedroom. Mine actually is.

Where you sit (or lie down) should be comfortable enough that both you AND your baby can remain very relaxed for an extended period of time. If you do not have support for your arms, you may experience fatigue holding your baby as he or she gets older and bigger. Your arm and back muscles will become stronger over time, as your child grows.

Pillows can be an easy remedy to this problem. Just make sure they do not have residue of highly-scented laundry soaps or fabric softeners on them and that they are placed with your baby's safety in mind.

Your baby should be comfortably reclined and snuggled in close to your body without being "suffocatingly" tight. Try to make sure the angle of the baby's head and neck is not awkward where it will eventually become uncomfortable and a distraction.

It will help if the location you choose is not overly warm or excessively cold. This is not always a factor you have control over, so just do the best you can for your circumstances and situation.

Let's face it, anything that takes your baby's attention off nursing — whether it be strong odors, loud or unusual noises, bright or unusual lights (including the increasingly rapid and irritating flashing of the images on the TV screen), uncomfortable position of the body, head or neck, shivering from cold, sweating from excessive heat, or inability to get the milk to come down — can jeopardize your ability to successfully breastfeed your child. You have to be aware of these factors.

It is understandable that you would prefer not to be rude to people who have stopped by to visit you and your new little one. If someone stops by to visit and there is going to be loud conversation taking place, however, you need to take a firm stand on excusing yourself (or asking them to excuse themselves) for the time it will take you to nurse your child. This is not really an area where you can compromise. It is critical — especially in the first several months.

Have you noticed in recent years how rapidly the picture changes on the TV screen? It makes me wonder if some of the problems with ADD and ADHD are not caused by a child's inability to process that much information in that rapid a succession.

Seriously try to avoid having your baby

nurse (or even rest or play) close to the TV set. It is worth thinking about. Especially on commercials, look past the edge of the TV while it is on and observe the speed of the images flashing in your peripheral vision. The speed at which the images change is hard for even an adult brain to process. This is something you can control, and it may make a huge difference in the long-term health of your child.

The voices and music on the TV also can create a negative environment for babies trying to nurse. The volume changes radically between scenes and during commercials. And all too often there is loud background music that muddles the voices talking on whatever type of program it is. This can have an effect on development of language in a child, as well. If you or someone else in the room is watching TV, make sure the volume is kept at a bare minimum if you do not have anywhere else you can go at feeding time. No compromise!

◆ ◆ ◆ ◆

Potential Adverse Circumstances

My younger son suffered from a spastic colon most of his first six months of life and endured considerable discomfort during feeding. There were times when the only place he could nurse satisfactorily was with me sitting in a chair at the dining table and him lying on the table top in front of me on a pillow. It sounds bizarre, but it worked!

There may be times when you have to use creative means and methods for nursing your child. Talk to your doctor, read, ask friends. Just do not give up. Keep trying until you find solutions to any problems that may come up.

Breastfeeding Your Baby: The Right Choice

A TASTE OF WINE
– PERHAPS NOT –
AND HOW ABOUT
THAT NICOTINE FIX?

Breastfeeding Your Baby: The Right Choice

10

To Wine or Not To Wine?

As much as I would like to, I am not going to go to great lengths to convince you not to drink alcohol while you are nursing, even though I personally believe you should avoid it completely. Hopefully you have listened to the advice of the "experts" and abstained while you were pregnant.

There are those who advocate drinking a glass of wine to help your milk come down. It is in the list of suggestions in many breastfeeding books and online texts. The theory is that it relaxes you. The problem is that your baby may be consuming alcohol, in trace amounts, which is controversial and could be risky.

If you are consistently using the ultra-warm washcloth method, there really should be no need for any other methods or means by which to get your milk to come down. I found the "secret strategy" to work 100% of the time. There is always the possibility that what worked for me and others will not work for you. No one method works for every person and every circumstance.

If, for reasons of your own, you feel strongly about being able to drink very small amounts of alcohol while you are nursing your baby, you will want to do some serious research on possible adverse effects of consumption of alcohol during breastfeeding a child before you open that first bottle or can. When in doubt, take the "safe route" and abstain.

♦ ♦ ♦ ♦

All Nicotine is Bad For Babies!

In states where smoking is still permitted in public places, you will want to make sure you avoid those areas, if at all possible. Second hand smoke (or first hand, for Mom) is an absolute "no-no" for pregnant and nursing mothers.

Exposing either you or your baby to second hand smoke is risky. I know it can be difficult to avoid when you have friends and relatives (or maybe even a spouse) who smoke. Even the amount of smoke that is absorbed into clothing can have a negative effect on the lungs of a developing infant. I cannot overemphasize the necessity to stay away from tobacco smoke!

Especially in winter when people wear their coats and smoke in their cars, you may be able to smell a smoker from 20 feet away because of what absorbs into their clothing and hair. Please do not ever take your infant in a car with someone who is smoking (or has been smoking recently). Between what absorbs into the upholstery, carpet, and headliner, the level of toxins in a car that people regularly smoke in can be very high and very dangerous to your little one.

Sometimes the results of exposure of an infant to second-hand smoke will not appear for years (like when your 12-year-old starts to play football and has to carry a prescription inhaler so he can breathe while participating in heavy physical activity), so you cannot count on the idea that your baby appears to be healthy now so, therefore, exposure to cigarette smoke must not be adversely affecting him or her.

I am assuming that if you are concerned about all of the other "natural" and environmental factors discussed in this book, you do NOT smoke yourself. If you do, you MUST quit today, for both you and your baby. This is not optional! Toxins in your blood are toxins in your baby's blood, both in the womb and through your breast milk. And toxins in the air are toxins in your baby's tiny, vulnerable developing lungs and respiratory system.

Do your baby (and you) a favor and totally avoid both alcohol and tobacco, if possible.

REST FOR THE WEARY MOM

Breastfeeding Your Baby: The Right Choice

11

The Dreaded Sleep Robber

This new adventure you are on, called parenting, will probably rob you of a lot of sleep during the first six months, although that varies with every child. After the initial "break-in period," it is usually about the time they start to date and drive that the sleepless nights begin to reoccur (with the exception of an occasional illness that keeps you up all night).

Nursing babies can commonly take in milk every two hours; and though you may go right back to sleep when you are finished nursing at night, you will still have interrupted night sleep for an extended period of time, depending on how long you continue breastfeeding.

It seems reasonable that this is one of the reasons why God created us to wake up frequently in the night toward the end of our pregnancies (often to go to the bathroom). Our bodies are, perhaps, being prepared to handle interrupted sleep for an extended period of time.

It is critical that while you are a nursing mother, you get as much rest as possible, because your milk production will depend somewhat on the amount of rest your body gets. All new moms get fatigued at times. If you get overly fatigued, it can have an adverse effect on your milk supply.

Keep your activities, exercise, and household chores at a moderate level, especially in the first few weeks, so that your body can heal and function properly, and so that you can produce sweet, perfect sustenance for your baby.

There are, indeed, families that are blessed with a baby who sleeps through the night most of their early lives, but this is not generally the "norm."

◆ ◆ ◆ ◆

The Cranky Caregiver – Not Me!

Beyond the milk production factor, a lack of rest can tend to make anyone "cranky;" and cranky people do not deal well with "demanding" babies. (All babies are demanding because they are created completely helpless and cannot provide any part of their own care).

When cranky people start expecting babies to not act like babies, bad things sometimes happen. We all fool ourselves into thinking that we could never be the mom yelling at a totally innocent infant at 3 a.m. It is important that we recognize when we are becoming over-fatigued and take steps to alleviate the potential for a loss of emotional control. This aspect of parenting is not always in our control; but the alternative to dealing calmly and wisely, with a cranky parent caring for a fussy infant or toddler, is disaster.

With your first child, you can often take naps during the day while your child naps — in some cases, every time your child naps. Please make sure you take advantage of each of these opportunities when it is offered to you. If you need to rearrange your schedule to accomplish this, then I highly recommend doing so. A nursing mom cannot get too much rest.

If you are a mom with more than one child, you probably already know that the ability to nap frequently is not going to be the same with the 2nd or 3rd or 4th child unless you have in-house help during the day. Hopefully, there will be at least a few occasions when your toddler is napping at the same time your freshly-fed infant ZZZZs off.

It is in the best interest of both you and your baby if you will commit to take advantage of opportunities every time they are offered to you.

It may also be possible to arrange with your spouse, parents, friends or church family to watch your older child(ren) at times when you are feeling extra fatigued and in jeopardy of compromising your milk supply because of lack of rest. It would be truly sad if your milk production tanked after all of your hard work, simply because you did not take advantage of the resources available to you in a time of critical need.

PLEASE DO NOT LET YOURSELF BE TEMPTED TO QUIT TOO SOON

Breastfeeding Your Baby: The Right Choice

12

Sometimes moms breastfeed for only a few weeks or a few months and then abandon their effort because of inconvenience or schedule changes or any of a number of variable factors.

You can expect each of your children to be different; and your family's financial and other circumstances may change from one child to another, as well.

I would encourage you to continue breastfeeding as long as possible — my younger son actually was still nursing at naptime when he was 3 years old. There was little milk involved at that point — it was more an issue of being a "pacifier" and a sure way to get him to sleep for his nap. When I needed rest, it seemed like the perfect solution to me; and I have not ever been able to discern that it did him any harm! (he is 23 at the time of this update)

No one is going to find fault with you if

you stop nursing your child WAY before age three, but you owe it to your child to give him or her the best possible advantage to start life out healthy and happy.

Statistics show that the longer a mother can nurse her child, the better it is for the child. The baby gets your immune protection, gets food specifically and perfectly designed for human babies, and you can continue to provide breast milk as a supplement to your baby's diet long after solid food is introduced and incorporated into the diet routine.

At the appropriate time, you will want to gradually add soft foods, then work your child into solid foods as directed by your doctor. If you can completely avoid supplementing with formula during this process, I personally believe your child will be better for it.

The risk of developing allergies or absorbing toxins from formula served in a bottle are real, in my opinion, and should be avoided unless there is no other acceptable solution.

If breastfeeding your child through at least the first year heads off even one possible future health issue, how can that not be worth the effort?

$$\blacklozenge \quad \blacklozenge \quad \blacklozenge \quad \blacklozenge$$

Circumstances Totally "Beyond Your Control"

It is virtually impossible for a child who cannot breathe through his nose to suckle, regardless of whether the source is a breast or a bottle.

Unfortunately, my oldest son caught a nasty cold when he was 10 months old. He was having a terrible time breathing and sucking — his nose was stopped up and even my best efforts could not seem to keep it clear. He struggled for several days with breathing and nursing and finally gave up trying to suckle at all.

I have to admit that this abrupt ceasing of my baby's ability to nurse was emotionally devastating for me. He would not take a bottle, and he was too young for a cup. My production plant was in full swing and I could not seem to pump it all out.

With a concerted effort, however, he was able to get enough expressed breast milk slurped from a spoon until he could swallow it from a "sippy cup." Sometimes

God throws these challenges at us, and we just do the best we can with the information, knowledge and insight we have.

Looking back (they say hindsight is always 20/20), I am almost sure there must have been a way to resolve the situation. If I had to do it again, I absolutely would try harder to find a solution to continue breastfeeding for at least another couple of months.

In my "ignorance," as a new mother with somewhat limited knowledge, I very likely "gave up" before I should have.

With the core issue, in my case, being that a baby simply cannot physically suckle if he cannot breathe through his nose, I could not see any solution at the time because I could not seem to get his nose and sinuses clear and keep them clear long enough for him to nurse. Maybe a nasal wash would have helped. Things I know now would have helped! I should have asked more questions and sought more information.

If something like this happens to you, be sure to consult your doctor or other medical practitioner immediately for possible solutions. The ability to continue breastfeeding for more than 10 months, in my opinion, is highly important. Ideally, I believe a full year is optimum.

My younger son had no such problems. He was a toddler before he gave up the "habit." Both boys grew up to be healthy adults, though. Neither has any allergies, food or otherwise; and neither has had serious illnesses to date (both in their twenties).

I certainly would not nurse any less than six months unless circumstances totally prevent it — and a year or more is better.

This is your child's life and future we are discussing, and the length of time consuming breast milk can be a factor in long-term health of your child.

Breastfeeding Your Baby: The Right Choice

THE FEW REAL "CONS"

Breastfeeding Your Baby: The Right Choice

13

Yes, There are Cons to Every Viewpoint

I could not fairly present this "argument" without at least including a brief sketch of the few "cons" that come along with a family's commitment to breastfeeding. After all, the idea behind writing (and reading) a book of this type is making an informed choice that will be in the best interest of your child and that will work for your whole family.

♦ ♦ ♦ ♦

The Sole Provider – You, Yourself and You

Unless you pump or express your milk and have bottles available for your spouse (or someone else) to feed the baby, you alone will be responsible for feedings 24/7/365. Formula feeding, with all of its "downsides" does allow for a helpful spouse or other family member to take a share of the responsibility. Stating this does NOT mean that I advocate that anyone who can breastfeed should not do so for that reason.

If you choose to breastfeed during the day and have your husband formula feed at night, I can almost guarantee that your milk production will suffer, sooner than later, and eventually become completely inadequate, just as though you were weaning your child.

Not feeding from the breast, during ANY time that you feed formula from a bottle, signals your built-in production plant that you do not need as much milk, and production slows down automatically. Once you allow production to get on a downhill slide, it is very difficult to recover it. (It can be brought back to full production in most cases, though. You just have to be dedicated and persistent.)

An alternate solution to using formula for "respite" would be to express or pump your own milk and have your husband feed the baby at night using sterile glass bottles with warmed breast milk in them. Keep in mind that this, too, can actually reduce your production, especially in times of growth spurts, because you generally do not get quite as much milk out on your own as your baby takes out. I have talked with women who were quite successful with pumping milk for night feedings and keeping up with production, though, so it may be worth considering.

Having your spouse feed the baby with your own milk definitely has less impact on your milk production than formula feeding at night does. Your milk production WILL probably be impacted, though.

I personally did not find the "all me" concept to be an issue. My husband worked in the oilfield and was gone from home two weeks of the month, anyway. I believed that it was well worth it to be committed to being the one and only "feeding specialist."

Bear in mind that, depending on his personality, the lack of opportunity for your spouse to be directly involved in the feeding of a breastfed baby can be an emotional issue for him, especially early on. You should make sure that "Dad" has ample opportunities to snuggle with you and baby while you are nursing, if at all possible.

There are plenty of other opportunities for "Dad" to be involved in nurturing of a baby besides feeding time. Take care to involve your husband as much as he wants to be involved, and always be sensitive to his need to actively be a father to his child.

I have even seen T-shirts designed for dads that express their support for breastfeeding as the best choice for their sons and daughters. And I know there are "support groups" for dads that provide emotional tools and resources for such issues.

My personal opinion on the new products designed to offer a dad a simulation of the actual <u>act</u> of breastfeeding a child is that they are questionable, at best. If the issue is to have the bottle at an appropriate angle, or to free up one hand by not having to hold a bottle, then such an apparatus may be an appropriate choice.

However, if the issue is providing a dad with "what nature has denied him," so that he can get as close as possible to "feeling" like a nursing mom feels while she's breastfeeding, then we need to talk.

God created women, not men, to breastfeed babies. Men are not being denied fulfillment of some inherent "need" by not being able to breastfeed a baby. God does not make mistakes.

A loving, nurturing father does not gain anything from a psychological standpoint by participating in an activity that is intended to simulate him actually breastfeeding his child like a woman would.

♦ ♦ ♦ ♦

The Soaked Provider – Oops!

Unless you are a nursing mother like no other, there will more than likely be times when your milk is going to "leak." You will occasionally find your clothes saturated and those around you eyeing you strangely.

For me, most of these occasions involved a dinner out with friends or family (and without baby) or a shopping trip that lasted longer than expected.

When you are away from your baby at the time your body is ready to feed him or her, even if your milk does not completely "let down," it can begin seriously overflowing. The longer you are away, and the more times your milk lets down, the more serious the problem will be.

This repeated letting down of your milk can be a very physically painful experience, and you should avoid it when possible, for your own sake. Having your milk let down multiple times without feeding the baby when you are out on a date with your husband or other event is an invitation to reduce production.

For some moms, this may be part of the "sacrifice" of breastfeeding. You may need to consider giving up most of your "social life" through the first year of your child's life, or host the social events at your own home, so you are available to breastfeed your baby when he's hungry.

You may find that even hearing someone else's baby cry in a restaurant or theatre, or snuggling up in a slow dance with your husband on a dance floor, will cause your milk to let down. It is worth your while to be well prepared. Depending on the fabric of your clothing, a major leak can be pretty hard to cover up — and pretty embarrassing to get through.

Nursing pads are widely available, so you generally should not have any problem taking care of this issue, as long as you have them WITH you. There were a number of times, though, when I went beyond what any amount of nursing pads could handle; and I learned my lesson pretty quickly.

Solution: Take plenty of supplies with you wherever you go, because you might end up having to use lots of them!

◆ ◆ ◆ ◆

The Picky "Eater" – Really?

You may have already noticed during your pregnancy that there are certain foods that do not agree with your baby. These commonly carry on into nursing. You will need to watch for foods you consume that upset your baby's tummy or bowels and avoid those once you identify them. They can change from pregnancy to nursing and can, at times, cause serious issues with your baby's digestive system.

Both of my boys had major problems with onions, garlic, broccoli, and anything spicy-hot all the way through my pregnancies and all the way through nursing. Although it created extra work, I did not want my spouse to "suffer" from this complication that did not directly have anything to do with him, so I cooked two pots of virtually everything — one with the seasonings in question and one without them. I knew it was only temporary and that it was ultimately worth the extra effort.

When in doubt, avoid highly-spiced and/or "exotic" foods. Consistently eat foods you know are healthy for both you and your baby and are not prone to upsetting either of your digestive systems. It would certainly be unreasonable for you to continue to consume foods you knew would upset your baby's stomach or digestive tract simply because you "like them" or you "want them." This is part of the commitment, it is not "all about you"!

♦ ♦ ♦ ♦

Shedding Your "Baby Fat" – Is It Time?

There is no doubt that you may end up carrying a bit more weight while you are nursing your baby than you would have if you had chosen not to do so.

It has been speculated, however, that nursing a baby can actually take the pregnancy weight off in a more consistent manner and ultimately get your body back closer to its "original condition" by the time your child is weaned.

If you have been careful to not pack on excessive pregnancy weight, you are probably in pretty good shape to begin with. Eating the healthy diet that goes along with breastfeeding will help you recover, especially if you have had surgery or a difficult delivery.

The big thing to remember is that your commitment to this "project" is limited to a fairly predictable time frame, and you will eventually be able to "do as you please."

With the exception of avoiding excessive fatigue and stress on your nursing body, there is no reason you cannot resume a strength training and/or aerobic exercise regimen, if you were doing so prior to (and perhaps during) your pregnancy. Just monitor your physical condition and make sure the physical activity does not interfere with your milk production in any way.

♦ ♦ ♦ ♦

Outweighed – I certainly think so!

It is obvious to me that the pros for breastfeeding your baby outweigh the cons, no contest. Hopefully you will draw the same conclusion when you have finished your research.

Breastfeeding Your Baby: The Right Choice

A FEW THOUGHTS ABOUT DIAPERS AND OTHER BABY-RELATED TOPICS

Breastfeeding Your Baby: The Right Choice

14

While we are on the subject of babies, we might as well devote a few thoughts to diapers.

I have to admit that my decision to use cloth diapers instead of disposables in 1983 had as much to do with conserving money as it did with conserving non-renewable resources and saving the environment. Although we could have afforded them, I just could NOT see spending that kind of money on something that was going in the trash. In some ways, I truly am my father's daughter.

The cloth diapers I initially purchased lasted all the way through one child and halfway through the second. Doing laundry is not my favorite activity by any means, but I truly did not mind the work that was involved with the choice to use cloth diapers. The monetary savings was in the thousands of dollars.

The only time I used disposable diapers was when we were on an extended vacation (seven weeks). Traveling 3,000 miles and staying with in-laws and other relatives in multiple states for nearly two months does not lend well to treating and washing cloth diapers. No doubt, it <u>could</u> have been done. But I wanted to enjoy my vacation! We factored the expense of the disposables into the cost of the vacation trip and gave ourselves a "break."

Not having babies of my own at the time of the update on this book does not keep me from having major concerns about the potential for toxins in the absorbent materials of disposable diapers, as well as the "housing" for the absorbent materials. The products widely available today in the form of "patches" and crèmes to infuse drugs and hormones directly into our bloodstream and tissues are solid evidence that virtually anything that comes in contact with our skin is likely absorbed into the tissue and bloodstream to some degree.

We owe it to our babies to minimize their exposure to all types of known and unknown toxins and chemicals that may be absorbed through their baby-soft skin. It is not like we don't have choices.

And the issue of generating almost mind-boggling amounts of waste that is not going to decompose in our lifetime — or our children's — should be of great concern, not only to me but to our society and our planet, in general.

I am in no way, form or fashion an "environmentalist," but I do believe we have to be responsible with our environment in areas we can control, and this is one of them.

♦ ♦ ♦ ♦

Breastfeeding as Birth Control?

It has been long contended that nursing your baby is an effective form of birth control. There seem to be plenty of studies and statistics to back that up, but I have personally known a number of women for whom it was not effective at all!

Bottom line, don't count on it.

Breastfeeding Your Baby: The Right Choice

IN CONCLUSION

Breastfeeding Your Baby: The Right Choice

15

When I was pregnant for the first time, I read everything I could get my hands on, and you will no doubt read at least several other books on the subject of breastfeeding your baby in addition to this one.

If you search the "information superhighway," make sure you consider the source as you read and study. Some information sources are much more reliable than others. And your doctor is always your final source of advice and counsel.

Obviously, not everything that is important to me will be important to you. And perhaps not everything that worked for me will work for you. However, what you have read here will give you plenty of "food for thought" and may steer you toward researching some of these ideas further.

It is my firm belief that this decision is important enough that I should share what I know and have experienced that may help you make the right choice: breastfeeding your baby from birth through solid food.

Advanced reasons for breastfeeding can include the idea that your child will be less likely to suffer from diabetes or be obese later on in his or her life and that you, yourself, may have less likelihood of being diagnosed with certain types of cancers in future years because you breastfed one or more children.

Although you, as the mother, are the one who will be required to make the most serious commitment in this decision, all decisions involving your children should ideally be made by husband and wife together. If you are a single mom-to-be, your decisions can be shared with your doctor, your close family members, or your church family.

If you do not glean anything else from this book, please try the ultra-warm washcloth treatment, even if you do not believe you are having "problems" with breastfeeding or milk let-down. It is just one more way to "hedge your bet" and give you a better chance to succeed in what will hopefully be one of the most rewarding experiences of your lifetime.

On a totally separate note, I want to caution you to take care in choosing those individuals who will care for your child when you are working, shopping, or away from home and your child for any reason. Child abuse, sometimes ending in serious injury to or death of the child, is more and more commonly perpetrated by an individual (either male or female) who is close to the mother – often a boyfriend and occasionally a paid babysitter. Protect yourself and your children, please!

The best evidence that breast milk is a baby's perfect food is that each of God's mammal creations is designed to feed its young its own milk. We are no exception. Happy breastfeeding!

TRAIN A CHILD IN THE WAY HE SHOULD GO, AND WHEN HE IS OLD HE WILL NOT TURN FROM IT.
~ PROVERBS 22:6 ~

Breastfeeding Your Baby: The Right Choice

ABOUT THE AUTHOR

"It's all about helping people," says Gretchen Slinker Jones of her writing, including two Christian devotionals, two books on résumé writing, a volume of poetry, a commentary on American politics, and other Christian self-help books.

Jones was raised and educated in the farm country of Southwest Idaho. She spent 17 years in Southcentral Alaska before moving to the "Inland Northwest" in the late 1990s, settling on the fringe of the beautiful Selkirk Mountain Range. The owner of a desktop publishing and business writing firm, Jones specializes in résumé writing for clients all over the globe. She has been teaching résumé writing for more than 20 years. Jones' freelance writing projects have included a weekly newspaper column for five years and a number of newspaper articles.

Most of Jones' titles are available on barnesandnoble.com, wordcopro.com and amazon.com. Search Gretchen Slinker Jones or G. S. Jones (Too Deep to Shovel) on these websites or in any internet search engine.

Jones writes poetry for adults and children, as well as children's short stories. Her poems, labeled as "Plain People Poetry," (including several that won awards and honors) are well received by widely varying audiences and are available in a "vocabulary and spelling" teaching format for both home-schooled students and public school classrooms.

Many of her readers enjoy following her Christian conservative blog at http://toodeeptoshovel.blogspot.com

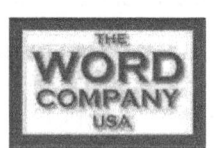

The WORD Company USA
www.wordcopro.com

Breastfeeding Your Baby:
The Right Choice

Covering topics such as how and why breastfeeding is the only choice and the right choice, portable and available 24/7/365, environmentally-responsibly packaged, priced right for even the tightest budget, naturally good vs. potentially toxic, and perfectly nutritious, this book offers the prospective nursing mother (and the father, too) insight and information that may be helpful in making the ultimate decision whether breastfeeding is the right choice for you and your family.

You have the opportunity to give your baby the best possible start in life. Your decision to breastfeed should not only help with early development, but may also influence the overall health of your son or daughter later in life, even into old age. What a precious gift you can give!

Jesus is coming again!